The Anti-Inflammatory Cookbook

Reduce Pain, Increase Mobility, Prevent Further Illness and Live a
Fuller Life eating Healing Foods!

Table of Contents

Introduction

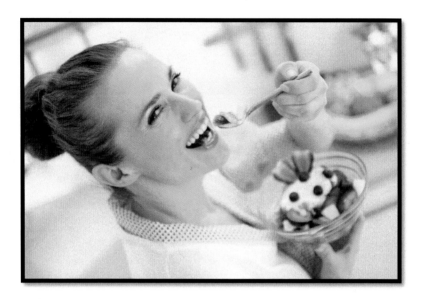

The human body is like a machine – it carries out specific processes in specific orders and every action has a scripted reaction. When your body sustains some type of damage or injury, it initiates the process of inflammation to help cushion and protect the damaged area from further injury while also starting the healing process. When inflammation persists, however, it can lead to a number of serious health problems. In fact, chronic inflammation has been linked to diseases like rheumatoid arthritis, Crohn's disease, and chronic active hepatitis. In cases like these, inflammation results in further damage to the body rather than healing.

In recent years, scientists and researchers like Dr. Andrew Weil have discovered a link between certain foods and inflammation. Eating these foods can have an anti-inflammatory effect on the body which can help to lessen the severity of certain inflammatory diseases. The anti-inflammatory diet is safe for people of all ages and it is a fairly easy diet to follow. In this book you will learn the basics about inflammation including its effects on the body and the different types of inflammation. You will also learn about the diseases inflammation can cause as well as tips about incorporating anti-inflammatory foods into your diet. Finally, you will receive a collection of twenty-five delicious recipes made with anti-inflammatory foods.

What is Inflammation?

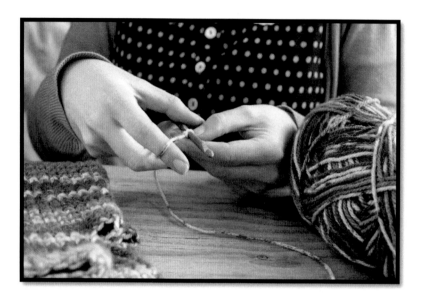

Inflammation is your body's natural response to trauma and it is a good thing, for the most part. When part of your body is injured or irritated, the tissues around it swell which draws blood to the area to help start the healing process. The word inflammation actually comes from the Latin "*inflammo*" which means "*I ignite*" or "*I set alight.*" Technically, inflammation is an immunovascular response and its purpose is to remove the cause of injury or irritation – to flush out necrotic (dead or dying) cells and damaged tissues and to being the process of repair. The most common signs of inflammation are redness, heat, swelling, and pain – severe inflammation can even lead to a loss of function in the affected area.

Stages of Inflammation

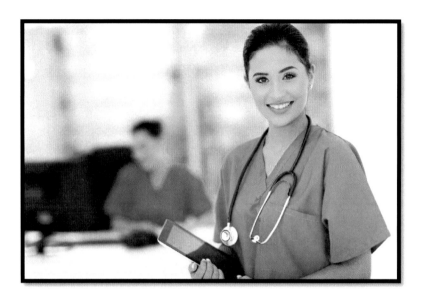

There are two types of inflammation – acute and chronic. Both forms of inflammation are closely regulated by the body because too little inflammation could lead to further damage while too much inflammation can lead to other health problems. Acute inflammation is the body's initial response to a harmful stimulus. When you cut or scratch yourself, the initial pain, redness, and swelling you experience is acute inflammation. Chronic inflammation is prolonged inflammation and it actually leads to a change in the type of cells found in the inflammation site. Rather than bringing plasma and leukocytes to the area to facilitate healing, chronic inflammation results in the simultaneous healing and destruction of the damaged tissue.

Acute inflammation typically lasts for a few minutes up to a few hours and it usually goes away when the injurious stimulus is removed. Chronic inflammation can least for months at a time, even years. In some cases, chronic inflammation is the result of failure to remove the injurious stimulus. In other cases, it results from an autoimmune response in which the immune system begins to attach healthy tissue. Some examples of acute inflammatory conditions include bronchitis, ingrown toenails and sore throat. Examples of chronic inflammatory diseases and conditions include asthma, tuberculosis, and rheumatoid arthritis.

Inflammatory Diseases and Conditions

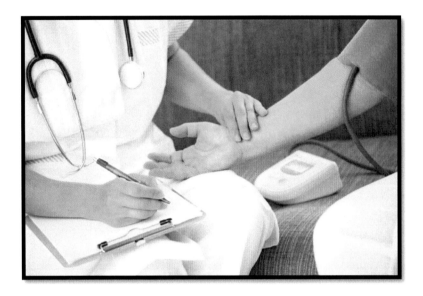

Chronic inflammation can be very harmful to the body because it results in the simultaneous healing and degradation of tissues. There are a variety of diseases and conditions which have been linked to inflammation, both acute and chronic. Certain studies have even forged a link between inflammation and obesity and various autoimmune conditions. In a study conducted by a team of researchers from the Pennington Biomedical Research Center in Baton Rouge, it was discovered that adult males with higher BMIs had increased white blood cell counts. Increased white blood cell count is a marker linked to an increased risk for certain conditions including coronary heart disease. While it is known that inflammation is linked to the development of heart disease and other conditions, still unknown is what causes the inflammation in the first place.

In addition to being linked to coronary heart disease, chronic inflammation has also been closely linked to autoimmune diseases. An autoimmune disease is characterized by the body's immune response to health tissue – in essence, the immune system mistakes healthy tissue for harmful pathogens and it begins to destroy them. Hundreds of autoimmune conditions include inflammation as one of their symptoms. <u>Some examples of inflammatory autoimmune diseases include</u>:

Crohn's disease	Addison's disease
Celiac disease	Type 1 Diabetes
Rheumatoid arthritis	Graves' disease
Fibromyalgia	Vasculitis
Lupus	Idiopathic pulmonary fibrosis
Psoriasis	Vitamin A deficiency

Aside from these autoimmune diseases, inflammation has been linked to a number of other conditions and health problems including:

Acute bronchitis	Tuberculosis
Acute appendicitis	Chronic peptic ulcer
Acute tonsillitis	Chronic periodontitis
Acute infective meningitis	Chronic active hepatitis
Acute sinusitis	Ulcerative colitis
Asthma	Chronic sinusitis

What is the Anti-Inflammatory Diet?

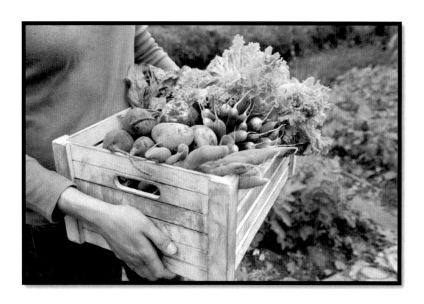

    The anti-inflammatory diet involves avoiding pro-inflammatory foods and eating more anti-inflammatory foods. Pro-inflammatory foods include things like processed foods, refined grains, certain meats and dairy products, high-glycemic foods, and saturated fats. Anti-inflammatory foods, on the other hand, include fresh fruits and vegetables, lean protein, seafood, nuts and seeds, gluten-free grains, legumes, and healthy fats and oils. Below you will find a list of both pro-inflammatory foods to avoid and anti-inflammatory foods to enjoy on the anti-inflammatory diet.

Pro-Inflammatory Foods to Avoid

Fast food	Wheat products
Fried foods	Soy products
Corn products	Gluten-containing grains

Vegetable oils   Alcohol

Refined sweeteners   Peanuts

Trans fat   Potatoes

Saturated fat   Honey

Fatty cuts of meat   Margarine

White rice   Ice cream

Starchy foods

Anti-Inflammatory Foods to Enjoy

Fruits and Vegetables

Acai berry	Collard greens	Lime
Apples	Currants	Orange
Arugula	Cantaloupe	Papaya
Asparagus	Cranberries	Peaches
Bell peppers	Garlic ginger	Pineapple
Blueberries	Grapefruit	Raspberries
Broccoli	Green beans	Romaine lettuce
Brussels sprouts	Guava	Rhubarb
Bok choy	Kale	Spinach
Cabbage	Kiwi	Strawberries
Carrots	Leeks	Sweet potato
Cauliflower	Lemon	Swiss chard

Turnip greens   Tomatoes

Nuts and Seeds

Almonds	Hazelnuts	Pistachios
Brazil nuts	Flaxseed	Sesame seeds
Cashews	Hempseed	Sunflower seeds
Chia seeds	Macadamia nuts	Walnuts

Meat and Seafood

Eggs	Sirloin Steak	Oysters
Chicken	Anchovies	Salmon
Duck	Cod	Scallops
Goose	Crab	Shrimp
Pheasant	Haddock	Tilapia
Quail	Halibut	Tuna
Turkey	Mackerel	Trout
Flank Steak	Mussels	

Fats and Oils

Almond oil	Coconut oil	Olives
Avocado	Extra-virgin olive oil	Grass-fed butter
Avocado oil		Walnut oil

Anti-Inflammatory Recipes

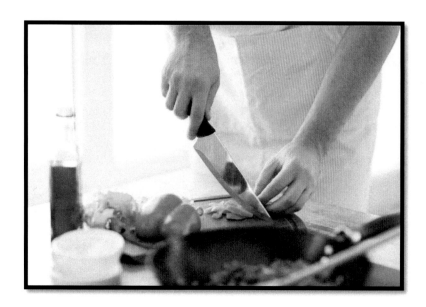

Recipes Included in this Book:

Cranberry Walnut Steel-Cut Oats

Easy Banana Pancakes

Blueberry Buckwheat Muffins

Tomato Spinach Omelet

Sweet Potato Cauliflower Hash

Herbed Turkey Burgers

Chilled Avocado Lime Soup

Strawberry and Sesame Spinach Salad

Grilled Balsamic Chicken Wraps

Creamy Sweet Potato Soup

Sesame Kale Chips

Cranberry Cashew Date Balls

Baked Cinnamon Apple Chips

Baked Sweet Potato Fries

Avocado Chocolate Mousse

Rosemary Roasted Chicken and Veggies

Grilled Salmon with Mango Lime Sauce

Thai Green Chicken Curry

Chipotle Lime Seared Scallops

Apple Glazed Duck Breast

Chicken with Puttanesca Sauce

Baked Swordfish with Tropical Salsa

Vegetarian Coconut Curry

Turkey and Broccoli Stir-fry

Black Bean Quinoa Burgers

Breakfast Recipes

Cranberry Walnut Steel-Cut Oats

Servings: 6

Steel-cut oats are an excellent source of dietary fiber which helps to regulate digestion and reduce your risk for heart attack and stroke. Paired with dried cranberries and chopped walnuts, this oatmeal is also loaded with anti-inflammatory compounds.

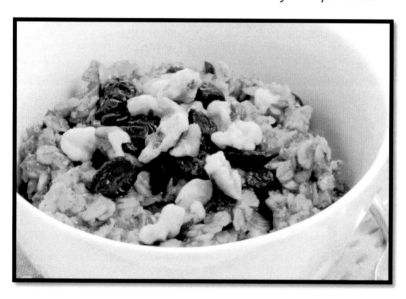

Ingredients:

1 cup steel-cut oats

4 cups water

Pinch salt

½ cup dried cranberries, unsweetened

¼ cup chopped walnuts

Instructions:

1. Combine the water and steel cut oats in a small saucepan.

2. Bring the mixture to boil over high heat then stir in the salt.
3. Reduce heat and simmer on low for 25 to 30 minutes until the oats are very tender.
4. Spoon into bowls and sprinkle with dried cranberries and walnuts to serve.

Easy Banana Pancakes

Servings: 3 to 4

Fresh bananas are packed with dietary fiber which helps to support healthy digestion. They are also a good source of potassium, vitamin C, manganese, and folate.

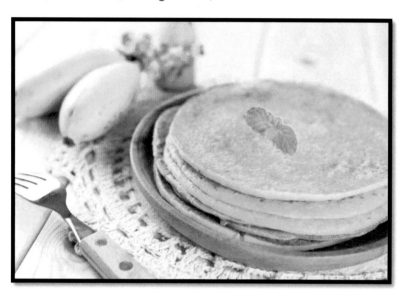

Ingredients:

4 large bananas, peeled and sliced

4 large eggs, beaten

¾ teaspoon ground cinnamon

Pinch salt

Instructions:

1. Combine the bananas, eggs, cinnamon and salt in a food processor.
2. Blend the mixture until smooth and well combined.
3. Heat a large nonstick skillet over medium-high heat.

4. Spoon the batter into the pan using about 3 tablespoons per pancake.
5. Cook the pancakes for 2 minutes or until bubbles form on the surface.
6. Carefully flip the pancakes and cook for another 1 minute or so until browned on the underside.
7. Transfer the pancakes to a plate to keep warm and repeat with the remaining batter.

Blueberry Buckwheat Muffins

Servings: 10

Even though it has "wheat" in the name, buckwheat flour is gluten-free. Buckwheat
is not only a great source of dietary fiber, but it also provides easily digestible
proteins and various vitamins and minerals.

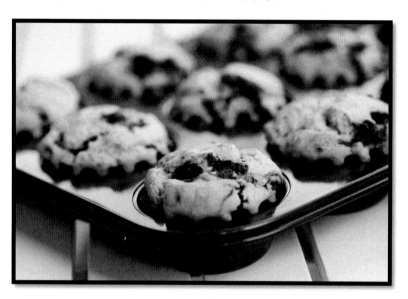

Ingredients:

1 cup blanched almond flour

2/3 cup buckwheat flour

1/3 cup ground flaxseed

1 ¼ teaspoon baking soda

½ teaspoon salt

½ cup unsweetened applesauce

¼ cup coconut oil, melted

¼ cup maple syrup

1 tablespoon apple cider vinegar

1 teaspoon vanilla extract

1 cup fresh blueberries

Instructions:

1. Preheat the oven to 350°F and line a regular muffin pan with paper liners.
2. Combine the almond flour, buckwheat flour, flaxseed, baking soda, and salt in a mixing bowl.
3. In a separate bowl, whisk together the applesauce, coconut oil, maple syrup, vinegar, and vanilla extract.
4. Add the wet ingredients to the dry, whisking until smooth and combined.
5. Fold in the blueberries then spoon the batter into the prepared pan, filling the cups about ¾ full.
6. Bake for 18 to 22 minutes until a knife inserted in the center comes out clean.
7. Cool the muffins in the pan for 5 minutes then turn out onto a wire rack to cool completely.

Tomato Spinach Omelet

Servings: 1

This tomato spinach omelet is an excellent source of protein and various anti-inflammatory compounds. Not only are eggs rich in protein, but they also provide significant amounts of selenium, vitamin B2, phosphorus, and vitamin A.

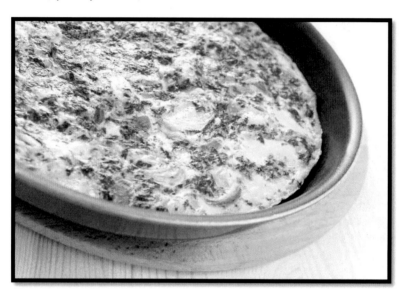

Ingredients:

2 teaspoons olive oil

1 clove minced garlic

1 small Roma tomato, chopped

1 cup fresh baby spinach, chopped

2 large eggs

1 tablespoon coconut milk

Salt and pepper to taste

Instructions:

1. Heat 1 teaspoon oil in a small nonstick skillet over medium heat.
2. Add the garlic and tomato and cook for 2 to 3 minutes.
3. Stir in the spinach and cook for another 1 to 2 minutes until just wilted.
4. Remove the garlic, tomato and spinach mixture to a bowl then reheat the skillet with the remaining olive oil.
5. Whisk together the egg, coconut milk, salt and pepper then pour into the skillet.
6. Cook for 2 minutes, scraping down the sides of the pan to spread the uncooked egg.
7. When the egg is almost set, spoon the vegetable mixture over half of the omelet.
8. Fold the empty half of the omelet over the filling and cook for 1 minute or until the egg is set.

Sweet Potato Cauliflower Hash

Servings: 4 to 6

This sweet potato cauliflower hash is loaded with healthy nutrients including dietary fiber, antioxidants, and various phytochemicals. Feel free to add a little kick of heat to this dish with a pinch of cayenne pepper or a minced jalapeno.

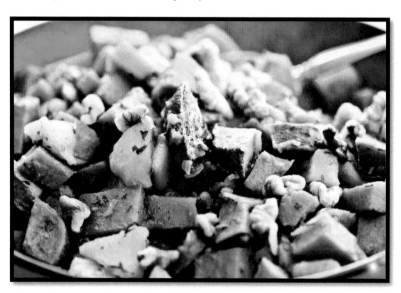

Ingredients:

1 tablespoon olive oil

2 large sweet potatoes, peeled and diced

2 tablespoons water

2 cups diced cauliflower florets

½ cup diced yellow onion

1 clove minced garlic

1 teaspoon chili powder

Salt and pepper to taste

Instructions:

1. Heat the oil in a large skillet over medium-heat.
2. Add the sweet potatoes and toss well to coat with oil then add the water and cover the skillet.
3. Cook for 3 to 4 minutes until the water has cooked off.
4. Stir in the cauliflower, onion, garlic, chili powder, salt and pepper.
5. Cook for another 5 to 6 minutes, stirring often, until the sweet potato and cauliflower are tender.

Lunch Recipes

Herbed Turkey Burgers

Servings: 4

Ground turkey is a lean source of protein, not to mention various B vitamins,
zinc, and selenium. In this recipe, ground turkey is flavored with fresh
herbs for a delicious and healthy burger.

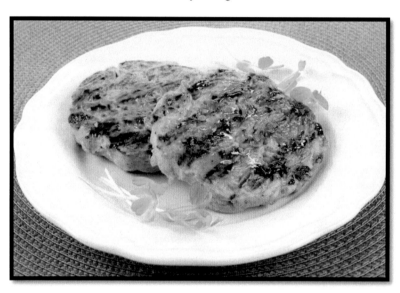

Ingredients:

1 lbs. lean ground turkey

¼ cup almond flour

1 large egg

¼ cup fresh chopped herbs, assorted

1 teaspoon Worcestershire sauce

½ teaspoon garlic powder

½ teaspoon onion powder

Salt and pepper to taste

Instructions:

1. Preheat the broiler in your oven to high heat.
2. Combine all of the ingredients in a mixing bowl and stir well.
3. Shape the mixture by hand into four even-sized patties, patting them to about ½ inch thick.
4. Place the patties on a broiler pan and broil for 4 to 5 minutes on each side until cooked through.
5. Serve the patties on toasted whole-wheat buns with your favorite burger toppings or serve them over a bed of lettuce.

Chilled Avocado Lime Soup

Servings: 6

Not only are avocadoes an excellent anti-inflammatory food, but they are also a rich source of monounsaturated fats. Monounsaturated fats help to lower your bad cholesterol levels and reduce your risk for heart attack and stroke.

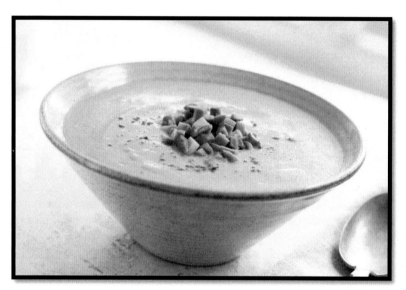

Ingredients:

3 cloves fresh minced garlic

1 small red onion, chopped

3 large ripe avocados

1 teaspoon salt

¾ teaspoon ground cumin

3 cups canned coconut milk, full fat

¼ cup fresh chopped cilantro

¾ cup cold water

¼ cup fresh lime juice

Instructions:

1. Combine the garlic, onion, avocado, salt and ground cumin in a food processor.
2. Pulse the mixture several times to chop then puree until smooth.
3. Add the coconut milk and fresh cilantro and blend well.
4. Spoon the mixture into a bowl and whisk in the cold water and lime juice.
5. Cover and chill for 1 hour or so until cold.
6. Spoon the soup into bowls and garnish with diced avocado and a pinch of cayenne to serve.

Strawberry and Sesame Spinach Salad

Servings: 4

This strawberry and sesame spinach salad is positively packed with anti-inflammatory foods. Not only is this a powerful anti-inflammatory recipe, but it is loaded with vitamins, minerals, and dietary fiber as well!

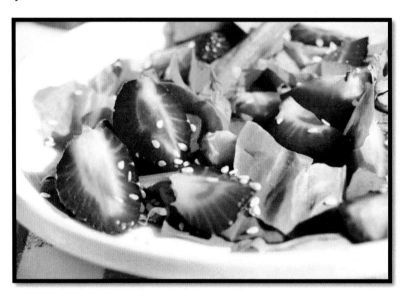

Ingredients:

6 cups fresh baby spinach, packed

1/3 cup extra-virgin olive oil

¼ cup balsamic vinegar

1 tablespoon maple syrup

2 tablespoons toasted sesame seeds

Pinch dry mustard powder

1 ½ cups fresh chopped strawberries

Instructions:

1. Divide the spinach among four salad plates.
2. In a medium mixing bowl, whisk together the balsamic vinegar, olive oil, maple syrup, dry mustard powder and sesame seeds.
3. Add the chopped strawberries and toss to coat.
4. Spoon the strawberry mixture over the salads to serve.

Grilled Balsamic Chicken Wraps

Servings: 4

These grilled balsamic chicken wraps are loaded with flavor and they are surprisingly easy to prepare. Feel free to load your wraps with whatever fresh vegetables you like and save some of the marinade to drizzle over the veggies before rolling up your wrap.

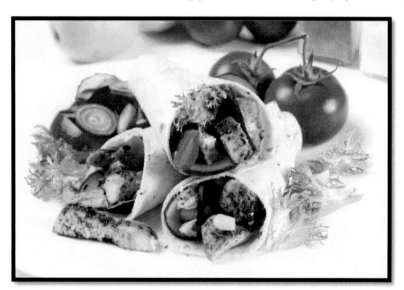

Ingredients:

½ cup balsamic vinegar

¼ cup chicken broth

1 tablespoon minced garlic

Pinch dry mustard powder

4 boneless skinless chicken breast halves

Olive oil, as needed

Salt and pepper to taste

4 large brown rice tortillas

1 large tomato, chopped

½ small red onion, sliced

1 ½ cups chopped romaine lettuce

Instructions:

1. Whisk together the chicken broth, balsamic vinegar, garlic, and dry mustard powder.
2. Pour the marinade over the chicken in a glass dish and chill for 1 hour.
3. Preheat the grill to medium-high heat and brush the grates with olive oil.
4. Place the chicken breasts on the grill and season with salt and pepper to taste.
5. Cook for 5 to 6 minutes on each side until cooked through.
6. Remove the chicken to a cutting board and let rest for 3 to 4 minutes then slice the chicken.
7. Lay the brown rice tortillas out flat and divide the chicken evenly among them.
8. Top the chicken with tomato, onion and lettuce then roll the tortillas up around the filling to serve.

Creamy Sweet Potato Soup

Servings: 4

In this recipe, sweet potatoes provide a mildly sweet and delicious flavor, not to mention powerful nutrients. Sweet potatoes are packed with vitamin A, vitamin C, potassium, manganese, calcium, and even small amounts of iron.

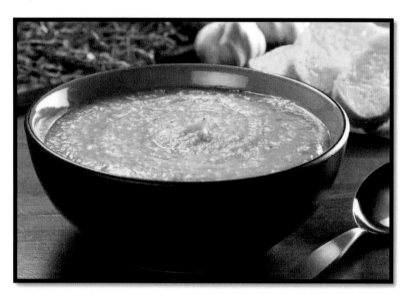

Ingredients:

1 tablespoon olive oil

2 large stalks celery, sliced

1 medium carrot, peeled and sliced

½ medium yellow onion, diced

1 lbs. sweet potatoes, peeled and diced

3 cups vegetable broth

¾ teaspoon dried basil

Salt and pepper to taste

Instructions:

1. Heat the oil in a Dutch oven over medium heat.
2. Add the celery, carrot and onion and cook for 5 to 6 minutes until tender.
3. Stir in the remaining ingredients then bring the mixture to a boil.
4. Reduce heat and simmer for 25 to 30 minutes until the sweet potatoes are very tender.
5. Puree the soup using an immersion blender until smooth then serve hot.

Dinner Recipes

Rosemary Roasted Chicken and Veggies

Servings: 4 to 6

This recipe for rosemary roasted chicken is surprisingly easy to prepare. Feel free to customize it to your preferences with whatever vegetables you have on hand.

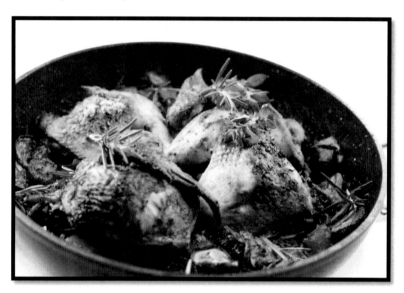

Ingredients:

2 tablespoons olive oil, divided

3 lbs. bone-in chicken thighs and drumsticks

Salt and pepper to taste

2 medium sweet potatoes, peeled and chopped

1 medium yellow onion, quartered

1 medium zucchini, sliced thick

1 cup diced tomatoes

2 tablespoons fresh chopped rosemary

Instructions:

1. Preheat the oven to 400°F.
2. Heat 1 tablespoon olive oil in a large skillet over medium-high heat.
3. Season the chicken with salt and pepper to taste then add it to the skillet.
4. Cook the chicken for 3 minutes or so on each side until browned.
5. Combine the vegetables in a mixing bowl and toss with the remaining olive oil and the rosemary.
6. Spread the vegetables in a 9x13-inch glass baking dish then season with salt and pepper to taste.
7. Place the chicken on top of the vegetables, skin-side-down.
8. Roast for 30 minutes then flip the chicken and cook for another 25 to 30 minutes until the juiced run clear.

Grilled Salmon with Mango Lime Sauce

Servings: 4

*In addition to providing plenty of lean protein and omega-3 fatty acids, salmon is
also a good source of vitamins A, E and D. In this recipe, tender grilled
salmon is topped with a sweet and tangy mango lime sauce.*

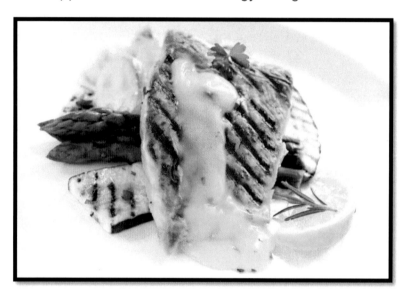

Ingredients:

Olive oil, as needed

4 (6 ounce) boneless, skinless salmon fillets

Salt and pepper to taste

1 ripe mango, pitted and diced

2 tablespoons fresh lime juice

2 tablespoons canned coconut milk

Pinch cayenne pepper

Instructions:

1. Preheat the grill to medium heat and brush the grates with olive oil.
2. Season the salmon with salt and pepper to taste and place the fillets on the grill.
3. Cook for 5 minutes then flip the salmon and cook for another 2 minutes or so until the flesh flakes easily with a fork.
4. Combine the remaining ingredients in a food processor.
5. Blend the mixture until smooth and spoon over the salmon to serve.

Thai Green Chicken Curry

Servings: 4

This Thai green chicken curry is loaded with flavor, not to mention healthy nutrients.
In addition to providing a wealth of anti-inflammatory compounds, the vegetables
in this dish also provide calcium, dietary fiber, and vitamin K.

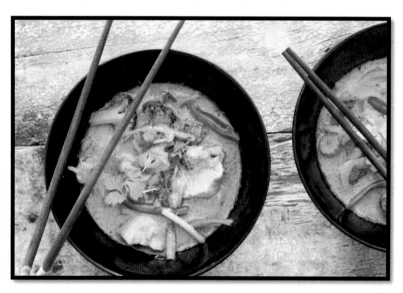

Ingredients:

1 tablespoon olive oil

1 medium yellow onion, diced

2 teaspoon Thai green curry paste

1 (14-ounce) can coconut milk

¼ cup chicken broth

1 tablespoon Thai fish sauce

2 cups fresh chopped broccoli florets

1 lbs. boneless skinless chicken breast, chopped

2 green onion, sliced

¼ cup fresh chopped cilantro

2 tablespoons fresh lime juice

Instructions:

1. Heat the oil in a large, deep skillet over medium heat.
2. Stir in the onion and curry paste – cook for 2 to 3 minutes until the onions are tender.
3. Add the coconut milk, chicken broth, and fish sauce then bring to a boil.
4. Stir in the broccoli, chicken, and green onion and cook over medium heat until the chicken is cooked through.
5. Add the cilantro and lime juice then serve hot.

Chipotle Lime Seared Scallops

Servings: 4

Not only are scallops an excellent low-calorie source of protein, but they are also packed with phosphorus, selenium, and vitamin B-12. Scallops are also a good source of choline which helps support a healthy metabolism.

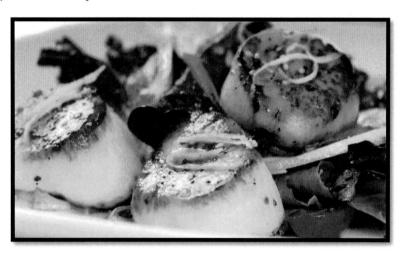

Ingredients:

2 tablespoons olive oil

¼ cup fresh lime juice

2 teaspoons maple syrup

1 teaspoon chipotle chili powder

1 ½ lbs. large sea scallops, uncooked

2 teaspoons coconut oil

6 cups assorted greens

Instructions:

1. Rinse the scallops in cool water and pat dry with paper towels.

2. Whisk together the olive oil, lime juice, maple syrup, and chipotle chili powder in a mixing bowl.
3. Add the scallops and toss to coat then cover and chill for 20 minutes.
4. Heat the coconut oil in a large skillet over high heat.
5. Add the scallops and cook for 2 to 3 minutes on each side until just cooked through.
6. Serve the scallops hot over a bed of assorted greens.

Apple Glazed Duck Breast

Servings: 4

Not only is this apple glazed duck breast rich in flavor, but it is also packed with healthy nutrients including protein, selenium and zinc.

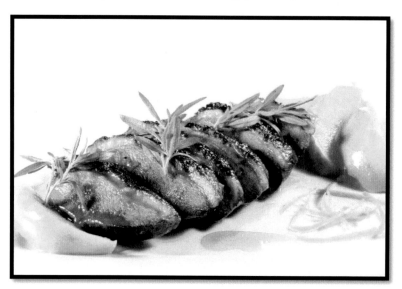

Ingredients:

1 small apple, cored and diced

¼ cup pure maple syrup

1 tablespoon olive oil

4 boneless duck breasts

Salt and pepper to taste

Instructions:

1. Combine the apple, maple syrup, and olive oil in a food processor and blend until smooth.
2. Preheat the oven to 400°F.
3. Trim the excess fat from the duck breast and use a sharp knife to cut a few slits in the skin.

4. Season the breasts with salt and pepper to taste then place them skin-side down in a large ovenproof skillet.
5. Heat the skillet over medium-high heat and cook the breasts for 5 minutes.
6. Flip the duck breasts and cook for another 2 minutes before flipping them back.
7. Spoon the apple mixture over the duck breasts and transfer the skillet to the oven.
8. Cook for 6 to 8 minutes until the duck is cooked to the desired level.
9. Remove the skillet from the oven and let the dusk rest for 5 minutes before serving.

Chicken with Puttanesca Sauce

Servings: 4

This chicken is easy to prepare and loaded with healthy nutrients. Everything
from the olive oil and garlic to the Kalamata olives and diced tomatoes are
packed with anti-inflammatory compounds as well.

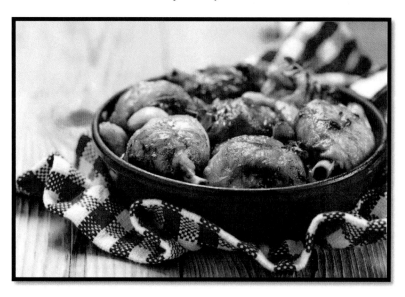

Ingredients:

2 ½ lbs. bone-in chicken thighs

2 tablespoons olive oil, divided

Salt and pepper to taste

2 cloves minced garlic

3 anchovies (oil-packed), chopped

1 (14.5 ounce) can diced tomatoes

¼ cup sliced Kalamata olives

1 tablespoon capers, rinsed

Instructions:

1. Preheat the oven to 475°F and season the chicken with salt and pepper to taste.
2. Heat 1 tablespoon olive oil in a large ovenproof skillet over high heat.
3. Add the chicken and cook for 2 minutes then reduce the heat to medium-high and cook for another 10 to 12 minutes until the skin is golden brown.
4. Transfer the skillet to the oven and cook the chicken for another 10 minutes.
5. Meanwhile, heat the remaining olive oil in a medium skillet over medium heat.
6. Add the garlic and anchovies and cook for 2 minutes, stirring often.
7. Stir in the tomatoes, capers, and olives then season with salt and pepper to taste.
8. Bring the mixture to a boil then reduce heat and simmer for 8 to 10 minutes until slightly thickened.
9. Flip the chicken thighs and cook for 5 minutes more until the skin is crisp and the chicken cooked through.
10. Serve the chicken thighs hot with the puttanesca sauce.

Baked Swordfish with Tropical Salsa

Servings: 4

*Swordfish is a low-calorie source of protein that also provides a generous helping
of omega-3 fatty acids. Paired with fresh mango and cilantro, this swordfish
also makes for a powerful anti-inflammatory meal.*

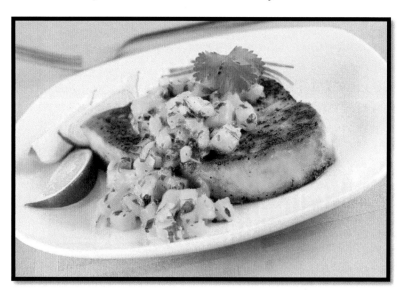

Ingredients:

4 (6-ounce) swordfish steaks

1 tablespoon olive oil

Salt and pepper to taste

1 medium ripe mango, pitted and diced

3 tablespoons minced red onion

2 tablespoons fresh chopped cilantro

1 tablespoon fresh lime juice

Instructions:

1. Preheat the oven to 400°F.
2. Brush the swordfish with olive oil and season with salt and pepper to taste.
3. Place the steaks on a baking sheet and bake for 10 to 12 minutes until just cooked through.
4. Combine the remaining ingredients in a bowl and mix well.
5. Spoon the salsa over the swordfish to serve.

Vegetarian Coconut Curry

Servings: 6

This vegetarian coconut curry is a powerful anti-inflammatory recipe because it is loaded with fresh vegetables like carrot, cauliflower and red pepper. Feel free to customize this recipe with whatever vegetables you have on hand.

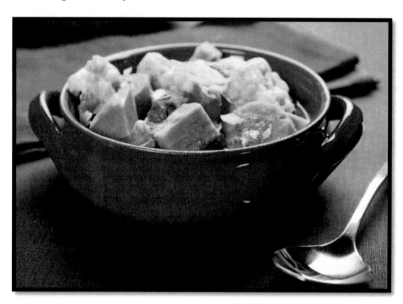

Ingredients:

1 tablespoon olive oil

3 cloves minced garlic

1 inch fresh grated ginger

1 medium yellow onion, chopped

2 medium carrots, peeled and chopped

1 cup fresh chopped cauliflower

1 medium red pepper, cored and chopped

1 ½ tablespoons curry powder

1 ¼ cup vegetable broth

2 (14 ounce) cans coconut milk

Salt and pepper to taste

Instructions:

1. Heat the oil in a large skillet over medium heat.
2. Add the garlic, ginger and onion and cook for 3 minutes, stirring often.
3. Stir in the carrot, cauliflower, and red pepper then cook for an additional 4 minutes.
4. Add the curry powder, vegetable broth, and coconut milk then season with salt and pepper to taste.
5. Bring the mixture to a gentle boil then reduce heat and simmer for 15 minutes.
6. Add the tomatoes during the last 5 minutes of cooking.
7. Serve over quinoa or steamed brown rice.

Turkey and Broccoli Stir-fry

Servings: 4

This stir-fry is loaded with fresh broccoli which is a great source of vitamin C,
vitamin K, B-complex vitamins, and dietary fiber. This vegetable is also
packed with anti-inflammatory compounds.

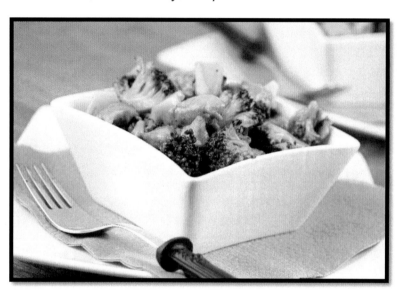

Ingredients:

2 tablespoons coconut aminos

1 ½ tablespoons orange juice

1 tablespoon rice wine vinegar

1 tablespoon maple syrup

2 teaspoons tapioca starch

1 teaspoon sesame oil

2 tablespoons olive oil, divided

1 lbs. boneless skinless turkey breast, chopped

1 tablespoon minced garlic

1 tablespoon fresh grated ginger

4 cup chopped broccoli florets

Steamed brown rice

Instructions:

1. Whisk together the coconut aminos, orange juice, rice wine vinegar, maple syrup, sesame oil, and tapioca starch in a small bowl.
2. Heat 1 tablespoon olive oil in a large skillet over medium-high heat.
3. Add the turkey and cook for 3 to 4 minutes, stirring often, until just cooked through.
4. Transfer the turkey to a plate to keep warm and reheat the skillet with the remaining oil.
5. Add the ginger and garlic and cook for 1 minute.
6. Stir in the broccoli and cook for 6 to 8 minutes until tender, stirring often.
7. Add the turkey back to the skillet and pour in the sauce.
8. Let the sauce cook for 30 to 45 seconds until thick and bubbling then toss to coat the turkey and vegetables.
9. Serve the stir-fry hot over steamed brown rice.

Black Bean Quinoa Burgers

Servings: 4

Quinoa is a gluten-free grain that contains nearly twice as much dietary fiber as other grains. It is also one of the most protein-rich foods available, not to mention a great source of manganese, magnesium, lysine, and iron.

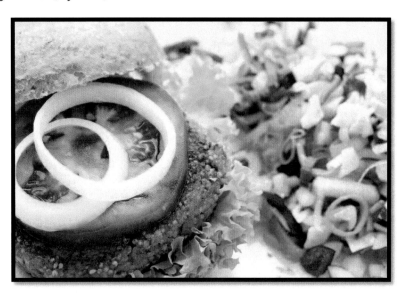

Ingredients:

¼ cup uncooked quinoa

¾ cups water

1 teaspoon olive oil

½ cup diced yellow onion

¾ cups black beans, cooked

1 teaspoon minced garlic

4 toasted whole-wheat buns

Instructions:

1. Combine the quinoa and water in a small saucepan and bring to a boil.
2. Reduce heat and cover then cook for 20 minutes on medium-low until the quinoa absorbs the water.
3. Heat the oil in a medium skillet over medium heat.
4. Add the onion, black beans, and garlic then stir in the vegetable broth.
5. Bring to a simmer and cook for 10 to 12 minutes until the liquid has mostly cooked off.
6. Transfer the mixture from the skillet into a food processor and add half of the cooked quinoa then blend smooth.
7. Spoon the blended mixture into a bowl and stir in the remaining quinoa.
8. Preheat the oven to 350°F and line a baking sheet with parchment.
9. Shape the quinoa mixture into four even-sized patties and place them on the baking sheet.
10. Bake for 20 minutes then flip the patties and bake for 10 minutes more.
11. Serve the burgers hot on toasted whole-wheat buns.

Sides and Snacks

Sesame Kale Chips

Servings: 4 to 6

*Kale is a low-calorie food that is loaded with healthy nutrients. A single cup
of fresh kale contains only 33 calories with 2.5 grams of fiber – it is also
loaded with vitamins A, K, and C.*

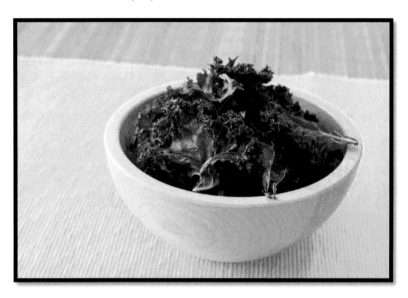

Ingredients:

2 bunches fresh kale

2 tablespoons olive oil

1 to 2 teaspoons salt

Instructions:

1. Preheat the oven to 350°F.
2. Trim the stems from the kale and tear it into 2-inch chunks by hand.

3. Toss the kale with olive oil and season with salt then spread it on a rimmed baking sheet in a single layer.
4. Bake the kale for 10 to 12 minutes until crisp and dried.

Cranberry Cashew Date Balls

Servings: 18 to 22

*These cranberry cashew date balls are loaded with dietary fiber and vegetarian
protein, all in a delicious and pop-able bite-sized treat.*

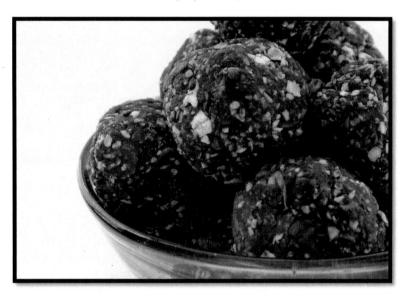

Ingredients:

1 cup raw cashews

½ cup pitted dates, soaked

½ cup dried cranberries, unsweetened

2 tablespoons almond butter

2 tablespoons coconut oil

2 tablespoons unsweetened cocoa powder

1 tablespoon maple syrup

Pinch salt

Instructions:

1. Place the cashews in a food processor and blend until it forms a flour.
2. Add the dates, cranberries, almond butter, coconut oil, cocoa powder, maple syrup and salt.
3. Blend the mixture until it forms a sticky dough.
4. Wet your hands then pinch off pieces of the dough and roll it into balls.
5. Place the balls on a plate and chill until firm.

Baked Cinnamon Apple Chips

Servings: 4

Fresh apples are rich in antioxidants, dietary fiber, and flavonoids. They are
also a great source of B-complex vitamins which are essential for maintaining blood and nervous system health.

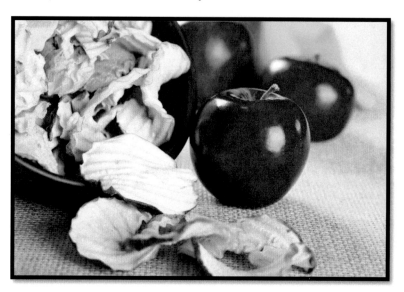

Ingredients:

3 large ripe apples

Ground cinnamon, to taste

Instructions:

1. Preheat the oven to 225°F and line two rimmed baking sheet with parchment.
2. Slice the apples as thin as possible and spread them on the baking sheets in a single layer.
3. Sprinkle the slices with cinnamon then bake for 1 hour.
4. Flip the apple slices and bake for another hour until crisp.
5. Cool the chips then store in an airtight container.

Baked Sweet Potato Fries

Servings: 4

Sweet potatoes are an excellent source of vitamin C and vitamin D, two vitamins
which are essential for a healthy immune system. Best of all, these fries
have just the right amount of crunch to them.

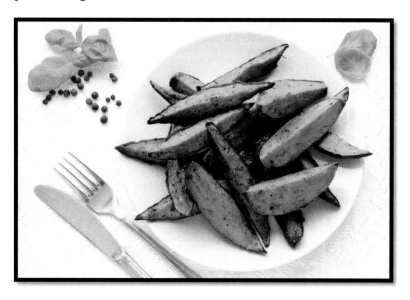

Ingredients:

4 large sweet potatoes, peeled and sliced into sticks

3 tablespoons olive oil

Chili powder, to taste

Salt and pepper to taste

Instructions:

1. Preheat the oven to 425°F and line a rimmed baking sheet with parchment.

2. Toss the sweet potatoes with oil and spread them on the baking sheet in a single layer.
3. Sprinkle with chili powder, salt and pepper to taste.
4. Bake the fries for 15 minutes then flip them and bake for another 15 minutes or until crisp.

Chocolate Avocado Mousse

Servings: 4

This creamy chocolate mousse is made with fresh avocado and sweetened with maple syrup. Feel free to dress it up with some fresh raspberries for added flavor.

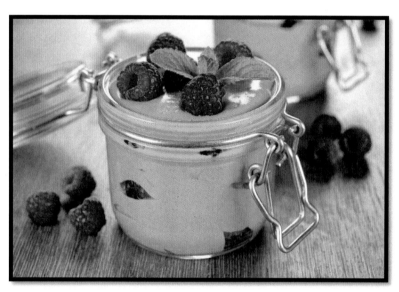

Ingredients:

2 large ripe avocados, pitted and chopped

2 tablespoons unsweetened almond milk

1 tablespoon chia seeds

1/3 cup unsweetened cocoa powder

¼ cup maple syrup

1 teaspoon vanilla extract

Instructions:

1. Place the avocado in a food processor with the almond milk, chia seeds, cocoa powder, maple syrup and vanilla extract.
2. Blend the mixture until smooth and well combined.
3. Spoon the mousse into dessert cups and chill for 20 to 30 minutes before serving.

Two Week Menu Plans

I have put together two week menu plans to get you started on your anti-inflammatory journey.

Anti-Inflammatory Meal Plan Week 1

Meals	Monday	Tuesday	Wednesday	Thursday	Friday	Saturday	Sunday
Breakfast	Cranberry & Walnut Steel Cut Oats	Blueberry Buckwheat Muffins	Banana Pancakes	Blueberry Muffin	Tomato & Spinach Omelete	Sweet Potato Cauliflower Hash	Poached Free Range Eggs with grilled tomato
Lunch	Turkey Burgers	Sweet Potato Soup	Grilled balsamic chicken wraps	Sweet Potato Soup	Strawberry and sesame spinach salad	Chilled Avocado Lime Soup	Chipotle Lime seared Scallops
Dinner	Vegetarian Coconut Curry with Caui-rice	Grilled Salmon with Mango Lime Sauce & Sweet Potato Fries	Turkey & Broccoli Stirfry	Rosemary Roasted Chicken & Veg	Apple glazed Duck Breast with Oven roasted Veg	Chicken with Puttanesca Sauce serve with Sweet Potato Mash	Thai Green Curry
Snacks	Kale Chips	Apple Chips	Cranberry Cashew Date Balls	Cranberry Cashew Date Balls	Kale Chips	Apple Chips	Chocolate Avocado Mousse
Make Ahead	Monday	Tuesday	Wednesday	Thursday	Friday	Saturday	Sunday
Prep for tomorrow	Make Muffins and Soup	Make Date Balls					Make Pot of soup and blueberry muffins.

Anti-inflammatory Meal Plan Week 2

Meals	Monday	Tuesday	Wednesday (FD)	Thursday	Friday (FD)	Saturday	Sunday
Breakfast	Blueberry Buckwheat Muffin	Cranberry & Walnut Steel Cut Oats	Sweet Potato Hash	Blueberry Muffin	Banana Pancakes	Tomato & Spinach Omelete	Sweet Potato Hash
Lunch	Sweet Potato Soup	Chilled Avocado Soup	Strawberry and sesame spinach salad	Grilled Balsamic Chicken Wrap	Sweet Potato Soup	Turkey Burgers	Rosemary Roast Chicken & Veggies
Dinner	Grilled Salmon with Mango Sauce & Oven Roast Vegetables	Thai Green Curry with cauli-rice	Chicken Puttanesca served with Cauli-Mash or Sweet Potato Mash	Baked Swordfish with Tropical Sauce & Sweet Potato Fries	Black Bean Quinoa Burgers with Sweet Potato Fries	Turkey & Broccoli Stirfry	Chipotle Lime Seared Scallops & Tossed Salad
Snacks	Apple Chips	Apple Chips	Sesame Kale Chips	Cranberry Cashew date Balls	Fruit salad (fresh!)	Avocado lime mousse	
Do Ahead	Monday	Tuesday	Wednesday	Thursday	Friday	Saturday	Sunday
Prep for tomorrow (optional)	Prepare Soup and more apple chips (if required)	Marinade chicken thighs	Make cranberry cashew date balls				Make soup for next week.

Conclusion

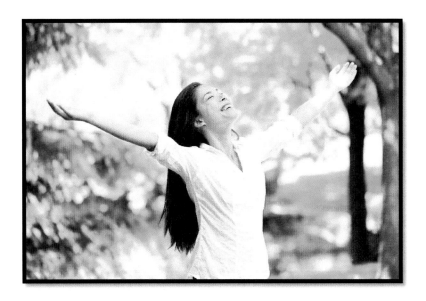

After reading through this book you should have a basic understanding of what inflammation is and what it does to the body. Inflammation is a natural response to injury or damage, but when it becomes chronic it can have a negative impact on the body. The key to reversing the effects of chronic inflammation lies in following an anti-inflammatory diet – that is, enjoying anti-inflammatory foods and avoiding pro-inflammatory foods. If you are ready to give the anti-inflammatory diet a try, follow the tips provided in this book and test out a few anti-inflammatory diet recipes from the two week menu included.